THE THINGS
KIDS LEARN TODAY

GENDER IDENTITY & EXPRESSION

VICTORIA RANGE – CARR

Dedication

To my spouse,

Thank you for allowing me to be a part of your healing process and personal journey. You've inspired me to see the world's youth in a whole new light. It is my honor and privilege to craft a tool to help families as they navigate the unexpected and unfamiliar terrain of parent-child relationships.

To Len Meyer, Gretchen Shelley, and Jill Reich, thank you for being my support system as I journey through my own set of unexpected paths. To have you all as colleagues and friends means the world to me.

Introduction

In a world that's ever-changing and increasingly open to conversations around identity, one of the most vital discussions we can have with young people is about who they are and how they express themselves. The Things Kids Learn About Today: Gender Identity and Expression was written to help facilitate those conversations in an informed, compassionate, and age-appropriate way.

This resource is not just a guide—it's a bridge. It's for parents who want to understand their children better, for educators and professionals working with youth, and for ministers or mentors seeking language that uplifts rather than alienates. Centered on truth, patience, and respect, this book equips adults to approach complex topics like gender identity and expression with openness and clarity.

Whether you're navigating new questions from a curious child or supporting a young person through their journey of self-discovery, this tool encourages meaningful dialogue rooted in love and learning. Together, let's create space for kids to feel seen, heard, and safe—just as they are.

How to Use This Book

Whether you picked this book out of curiosity, care, or a desire to better support the young people in your life — welcome. This resource was created with the intention of bridging conversations about gender identity and expression in ways that are clear, supportive, and affirming.

Here are a few gentle guidelines to help you navigate the pages ahead:

1. Read with an open heart.
This book is designed to meet you where you are—whether this topic is familiar or completely new. Approach each section with curiosity and compassion, both for yourself and for the young people you're supporting.

2. Take your time.
There's no need to rush. This book is intended to be read together by an adult and child together. However, you may feel more comfortable reading the book on your own first and then revisiting the text with your parent/caretaker, counselor, child or student, at a later time. Be prepared, some pages may spark deep conversations. That's okay. Pause, reflect, and return as needed.

3. Let the language guide your conversations.
The words and phrases used here are meant to model respectful and inclusive dialogue. Feel free to use them as talking points, journaling prompts, or ways to reframe your own thoughts and language. You'll also find terms explained simply so you can feel confident discussing them with others.

4. Use it in your setting.

This book can be shared one-on-one or in small group discussions—at home, in classrooms, counseling sessions, youth groups, or faith-based settings. It's flexible and welcoming to diverse beliefs and family values, while still affirming the dignity of every child.

5. Revisit as kids grow.

Gender identity and self-expression are lifelong topics. One's questions, understanding, and self-awareness may evolve—and so can your conversations. This book can grow with you, offering fresh meaning at each stage.

6. When in doubt, lean into love.

You don't need all the answers. What's needed most is your willingness to listen, learn, and walk together. This book is simply one tool to help you do just that—with love at the center of the journey.

FOR CHILDREN READING THIS BOOK

This book was written for you because you are the generation of openness. Generations before you weren't allowed to have social openness or legally protected self-expression. The world is changing. And while some people still resist the bravery it takes to be your own kind of wonderful, you have social and legal support for open communication and self-expression. I want to encourage you to be yourself, at all times.

I also want to encourage you to be patient with those caring for you, living around you and maybe even teaching you... because there have been strict rules in the past about conforming and adhering to social and cultural expectations. Those much older than you won't necessarily understand you at first. Maybe they never felt safe enough to speak up without shame about what others would think or believe. Maybe those in your community have been more conforming to the expectations of others than you prefer to be. Maybe they never had anyone to encourage them to own, embrace, and develop their sense of self. Either way, you should know that for generations, societal rules did not promote inclusiveness–there are some today, continuing in that pattern of thinking. So, consider yourselves teachers to the elders. Teach them with the same love, patience, honor, and respect that you wish to receive from them.

Most of all, remember this, no matter how unique we are, we're all in this together. That's what it means to be part of the LGBTQIA community whether you are Lesbian, Gay, Bisexual, Transgender, Queer, Inquiring, or an Ally. You are worthy of love, belonging, and the freedom to be exactly who you are.

FOR THE PARENT/CAREGIVER

This book is an invitation for you to explore communication with your child(ren) and topics that may have once been considered taboo or off-limits. It doesn't matter whether biological, grand, step, adoptive, or fictive kin.

The act of being willing to facilitate open and safe communication with children will lead to stronger relationship dynamics. Though it may seem difficult and uncomfortable at first, with practice, the process will become easier for everyone.

Open and safe dialogue between parents and their children facilitates the development and maintenance of healthy and strong parent-child relationships. It is also foundational for the development of youth as they transition into adulthood. While there are many tough conversations parents must have with their children, this book focuses on the topic of "Gender Identity, and Expression," of the overarching subject of Sexual Orientation, Gender Identity and Expression (SOGIE). SOGIE is the term used to reference how people experience and express their identities. What most people don't know is that everyone, regardless of age, religion, or culture, has an organic sexual orientation and gender identity. Using SOGIE language helps bring context to our individual experiences.

Many of us were raised with limited guidance or the flexibility to explore our thoughts, feelings, sexuality or gender identity. These parameters were often preset for us, and we were required to comply in very specific ways. In both my professional and personal opinion, these limitations muted our self-awareness and limited our self-expression. I believe it is to our advantage to change the pattern of stifling individualism by offering our children the time and opportunity to explore their feelings, thoughts, and perceptions and to openly share them with us, their caretakers.

In considering parenting practices over the years, and across generations, one of the reasons I believe parents limit self-exploration in children is that parents are afraid they won't know what to do with what their children bring to them. I'm here to tell you we don't have to discourage young people from talking to us out of fear that we may not know what to say or how to respond. An immediate response is not necessary if there is no immediate risk of physical harm to oneself or others. The idea that everything needs to be decided right now is not a fact. Think about it. We often feel pressure to respond immediately, but unless there's a risk of physical harm, it's okay to pause. Listening is enough.

Another reason I think parents have historically limited the nature of children to explore natural curiosity is the adage passed down through the generations that "children are to be seen and not heard." A healthier approach might be "there is a time and place for all discussions." This shift allows us to create a protected space for our children (and ourselves) when we just can't predict what they may want to talk about. In this manner, we still honor their voice. The former concept of seen and not heard stifles and limits a child's ability to practice conveying their thoughts and feelings. A child without practice in identifying and communicating their thoughts and feelings soon becomes an adult incapable of the same. So even though we may need to redirect a discussion to a safe place and time, it is imperative to make room for whatever a child wants to discuss, including gender and identity.

Take a moment to think about how communication was managed when you were a child. Did you feel emotionally safe to share your thoughts and feelings about things that were important to you? How did that make you feel? As a young person, did you ever feel physically and emotionally safe to go to a parent, caregiver or another adult to discuss anything of significance to you, like a secret crush, bullying at school, an assault by an adult, or abuse by a sibling? Consider how those experiences have shaped how you respond to your children now.

I know I'm asking a lot of questions, but I want to get you to remember your needs as a youth and consider how significant this is for your child to be able to communicate with you and have your emotional support as they develop their identity. Children of all ages need to be seen and heard as they grow.

Your willingness to listen, even when it's hard, creates space for your child to feel seen and supported. That alone can be life-changing.

FOR THE PROFESSIONAL

This book is intended to be a resource for youth, parents, and caregivers who would benefit from increasing their understanding and/or exploration of Sexual Orientation, Gender Identity, and Expression (SOGIE). It is also recommended for families learning to communicate about the Lesbian, Gay, Bisexual, Transgender, Queer (LGBTQIA) life experiences.

Throughout this book, the term SOGIE will be used to refer to the broad range of how people experience and express their identities. Everyone, regardless of age or background, has a sexual orientation and gender identity. Using SOGIE language helps us shift from thinking in terms of labels to focusing on personal experiences. This allows for more respectful, inclusive, and stigma-free conversations.

This book is ideal for parents, caregivers including foster parents, extended family, fictive-kin and professionals providing direct care and/or services to youth in residential facilities and other social service programs.

I hope this book serves as a resource for launching safe, honest conversations between youth and their families. These discussions can be guided compassionately by advocates like you, whether in counseling sessions or through independent reading.

I encourage the use of this book in professional and faith-based trainings, discussions, meetings and/or individual staffings to:

- provide opportunities for safe discussions in the workplace,
- facilitate professional exploration of self-awareness and personal bias,
- decrease social, cultural, religious, and institutional bias in the workplace,
- strengthen workers' ability to communicate and support youth in exercising their right to self-expression and their families, and
- increase the effectiveness of professional interventions, where SOGIE is a contributing factor to family dysfunction.

Above all, this resource aims to help professionals like you support youth and their families with empathy, clarity, and confidence.

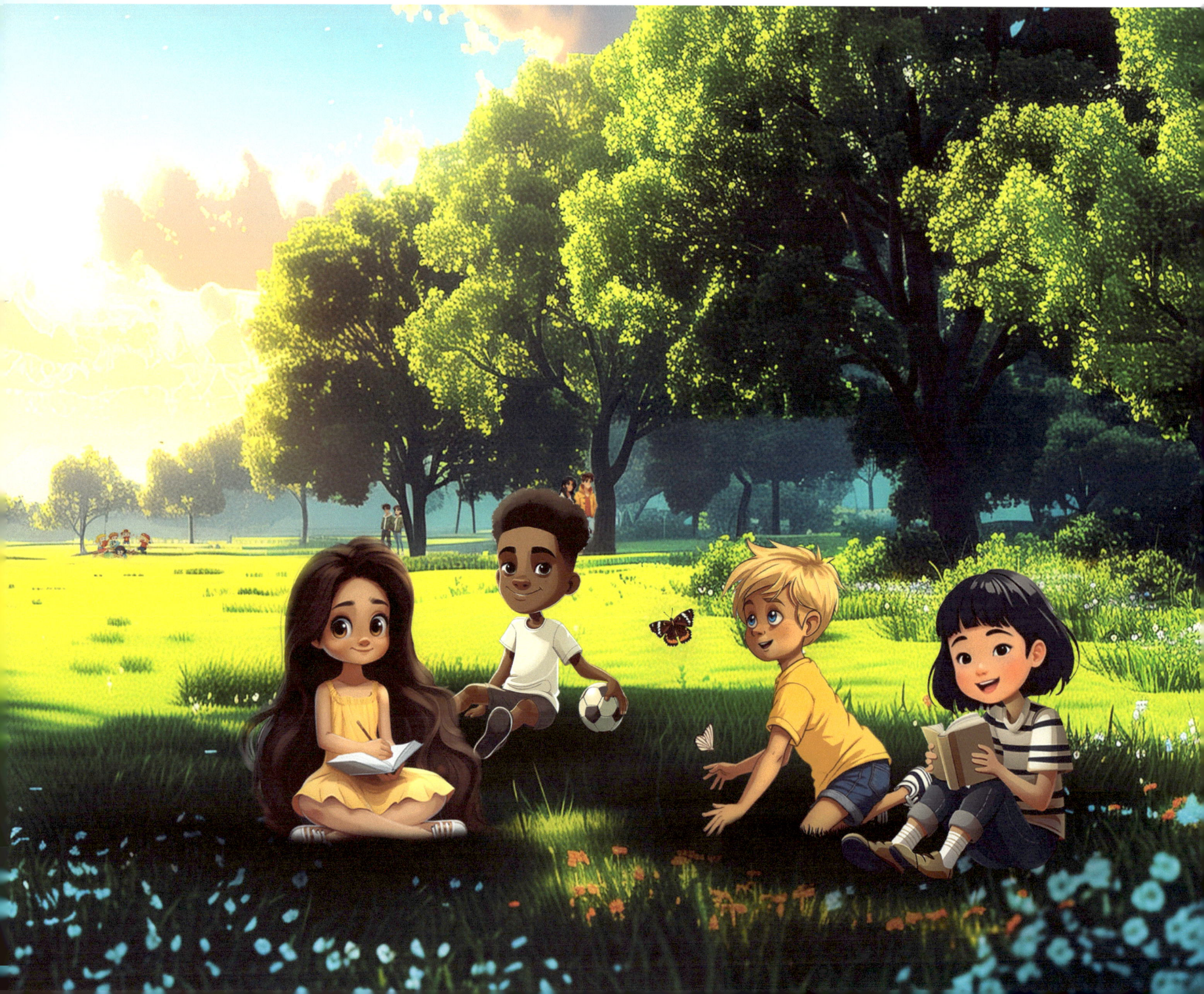

Today, children grow up so fast. They learn so much and figure out quickly who they are and what they want. It all happens in the blink of an eye, and sometimes, it can feel hard for a parent to keep up.

You'll see what we mean, as you learn more about Johnnie, Mare, Don and Ella.

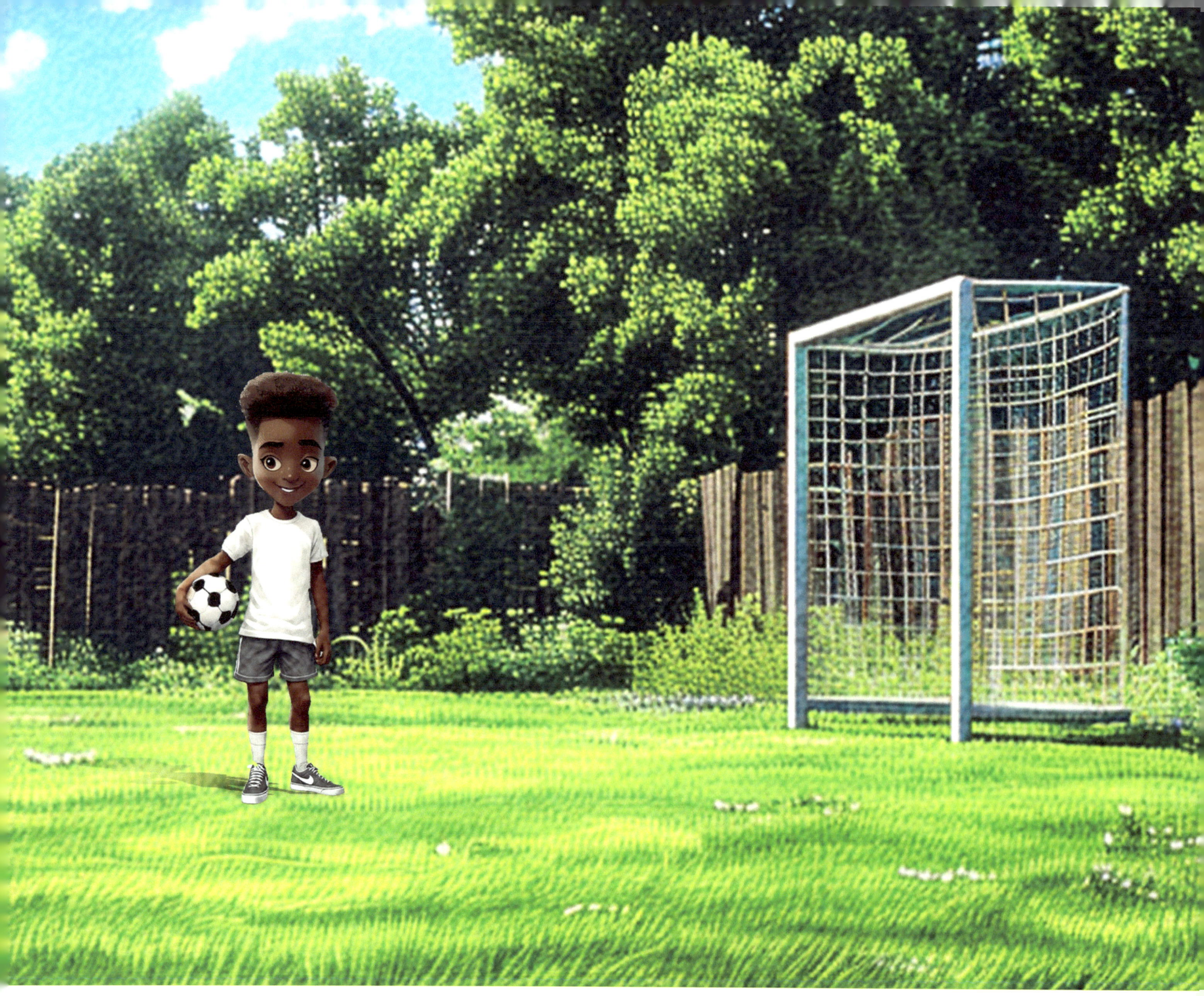

This is John. He is a male-born child, and he uses the pronouns he/him/his. He likes his family and friends to call him Johnnie.

Johnnie's favorite activities include playing soccer, getting together with his friends, and going to school. Johnnie gets good grades, has lots of friends, and his parents are very proud of his All-Star status. Johnnie meets all of his parents' dreams and expectations – even the ones they had before he was born.

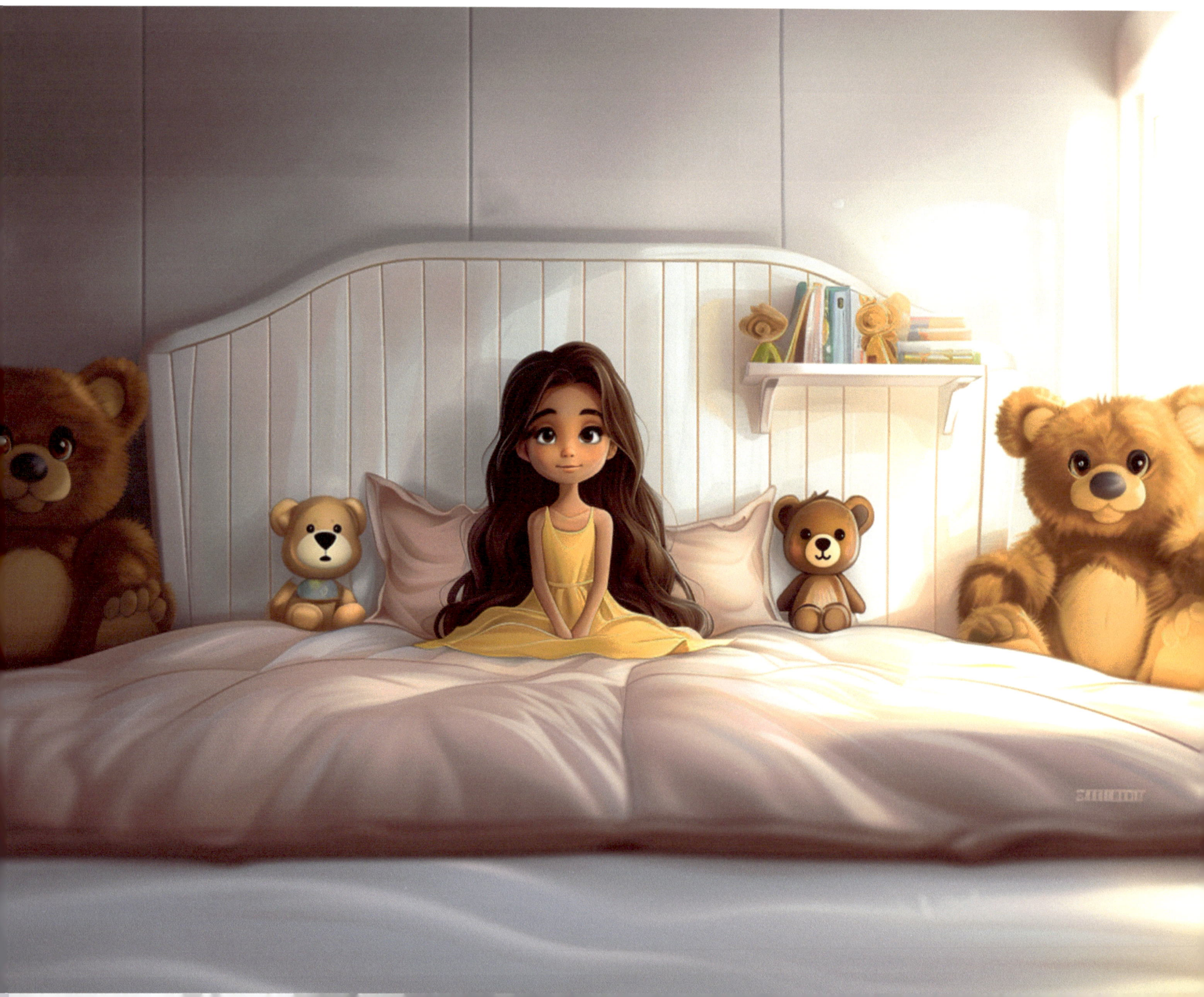

This is Mary. She was female-assigned at birth, and her pronouns are she, her, and hers. Her friends and family call her Mare because it is what Mary prefers.

Mare enjoys playing with her dolls, playing dress up, and putting on lip gloss. When she is in school, she plays jump rope with her friends at recess, and she is known for completing her homework before the end of the school day.

Her parents are extremely proud of Mare's ladylike demeanor and social skills. They often tell her that she is everything they have ever wanted and expected in a daughter.

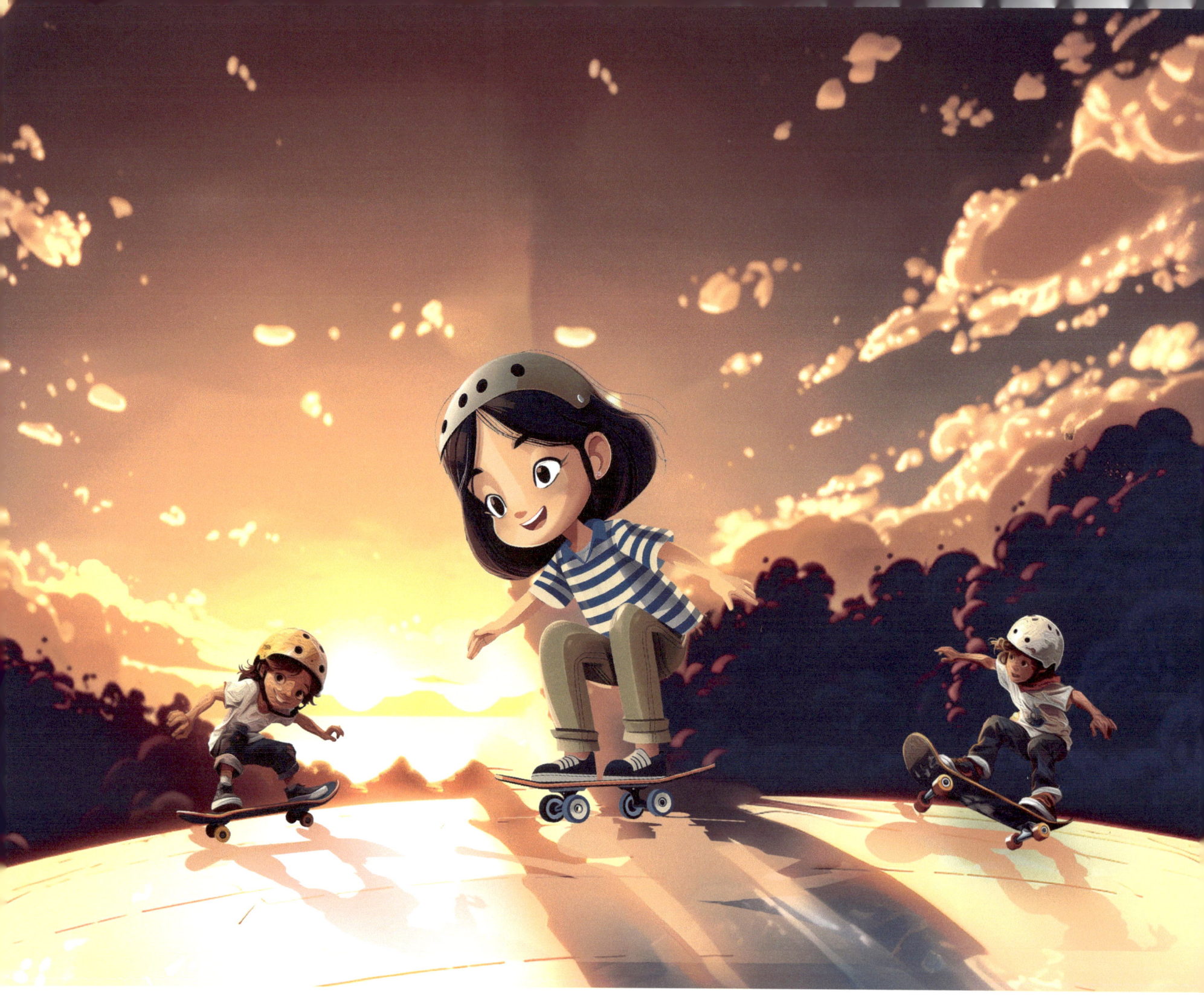

This is Donna. Donna prefers to be called Don. Don uses the pronouns he/him/his. While Don was assigned female at birth, he feels most confident in ways some people might say is masculine.

His hobbies include skateboarding in the park and hunting for frogs by the creek. Though female-assigned at birth, Don does not like to play pretend doll games with his sister but prefers football in the rain with his cousin Bobby. At school, Don gets good grades, plays basketball, and is always the star player, no matter the team he's on.

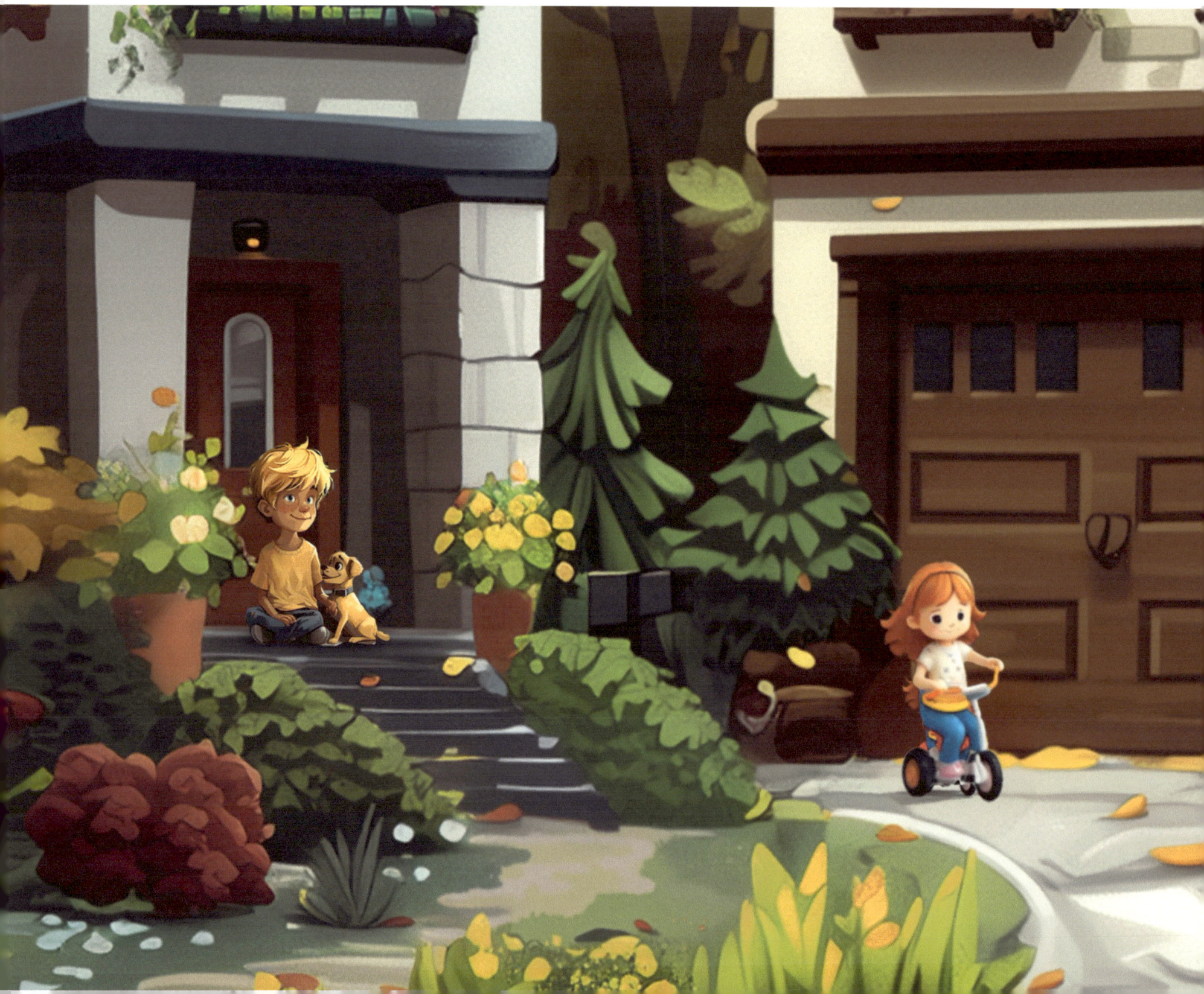

This is Daniel, male-assigned at birth, as you might assume at first sight. What you can't see is that Daniel answers to the name "Ella," uses the pronouns she/her/hers, and openly identifies as a girl. Daniel is very comfortable with expressing herself in ways that are traditionally considered "feminine."

One day when Daniel…I'm sorry, "Ella" was younger, she watched a movie with a character named "Ella." That character was very feminine, strong-willed, confident, and outspoken. Observing this character, Daniel (at the time) experienced a strong sense of connection and validation. From that point, Daniel was able to identify their thoughts and feelings about who he or rather, she is as an individual. That moment helped Daniel decide to be honest with himself and with others. He immediately told his parents about this experience. From that point on, Daniel used the pronouns she/her/hers and the name "Ella," and quickly began to blossom. From that day forward, like a caterpillar transforms into a butterfly, "Daniel," now "Ella," settled into a place of inner peace and calm. It was evidenced in her feminine expression and increasingly confident communication.

Daniel's parents always knew something was different about their little one. Over the years, they noticed that "Daniel," or rather "Ella," even as a toddler, was quiet and observant and did not communicate as other male-assigned children they knew. As their baby grew, what they saw and what they expected did not line up. They often worried that something was wrong. No matter how they tried, they couldn't put their finger on what was making them so uncomfortable about their observations. Needless to say, their child's declaration of identity brought both some resolve and some fear. Despite those fears, they supported their child's self-expression of gender and identity.

At times, Ella's parents had to ask how they could best support and love her – because they never expected to parent a male-assigned child whose self-expression reflected their mother's more than their father's.

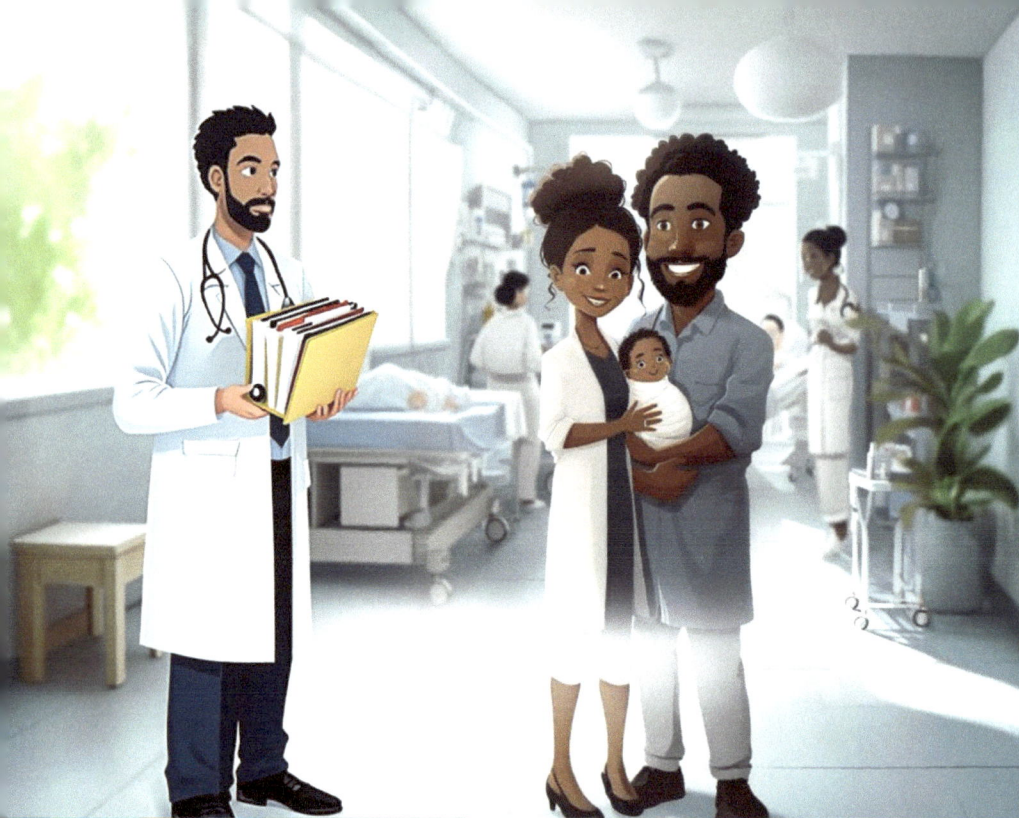

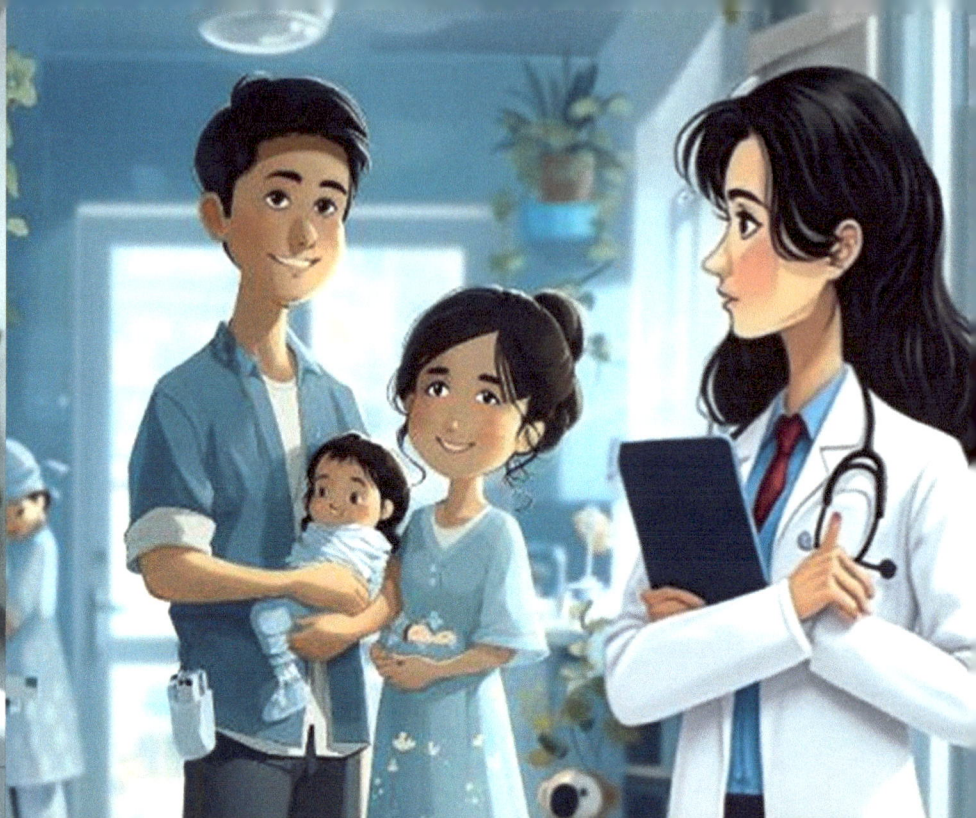

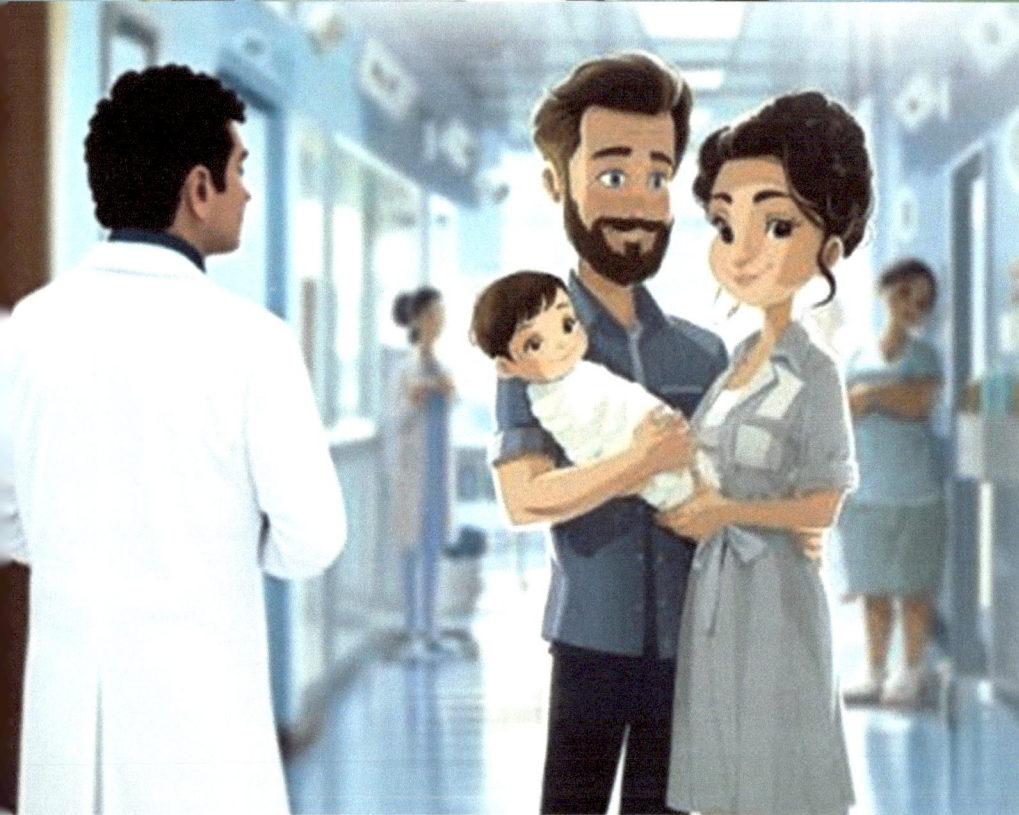

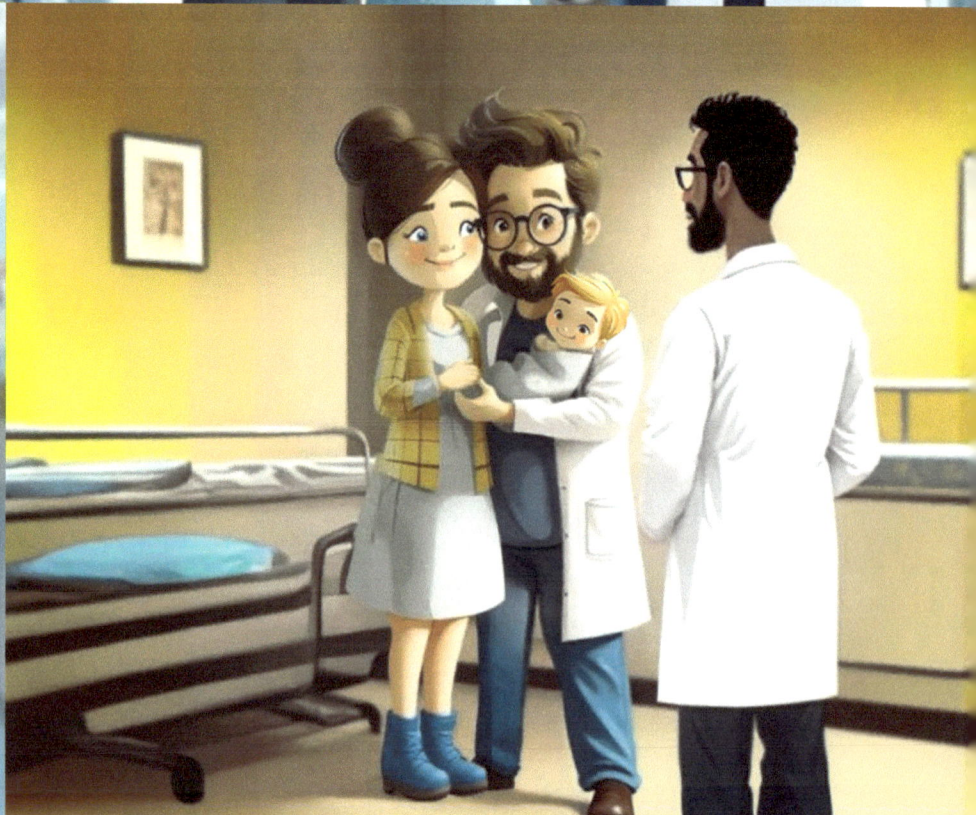

When John, Mary, Donna, and Daniel came into the world, they were babies just like us. They were healthy, strong, and loved. Before going home, the doctors gave each baby — and their mother a clean bill of health. Everyone smiled excitedly as their family was released from the hospital without any concerns.

The babies and their parents were ready to go home and begin their new journeys through life surrounded by love and possibilities.

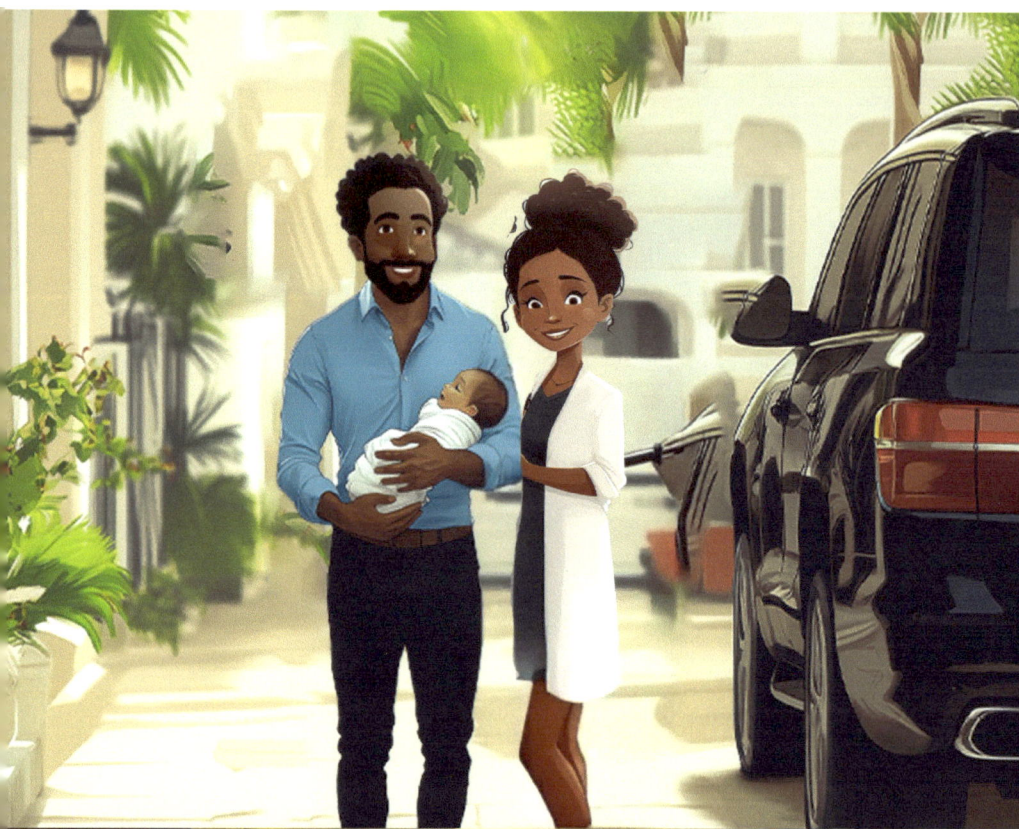
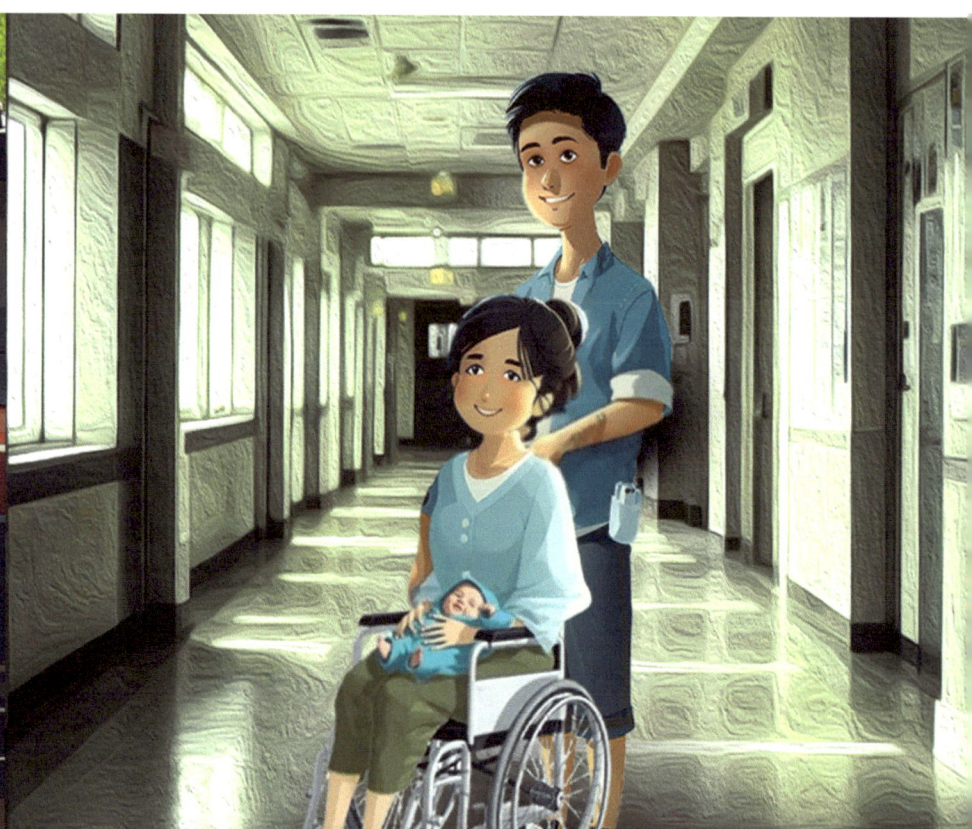
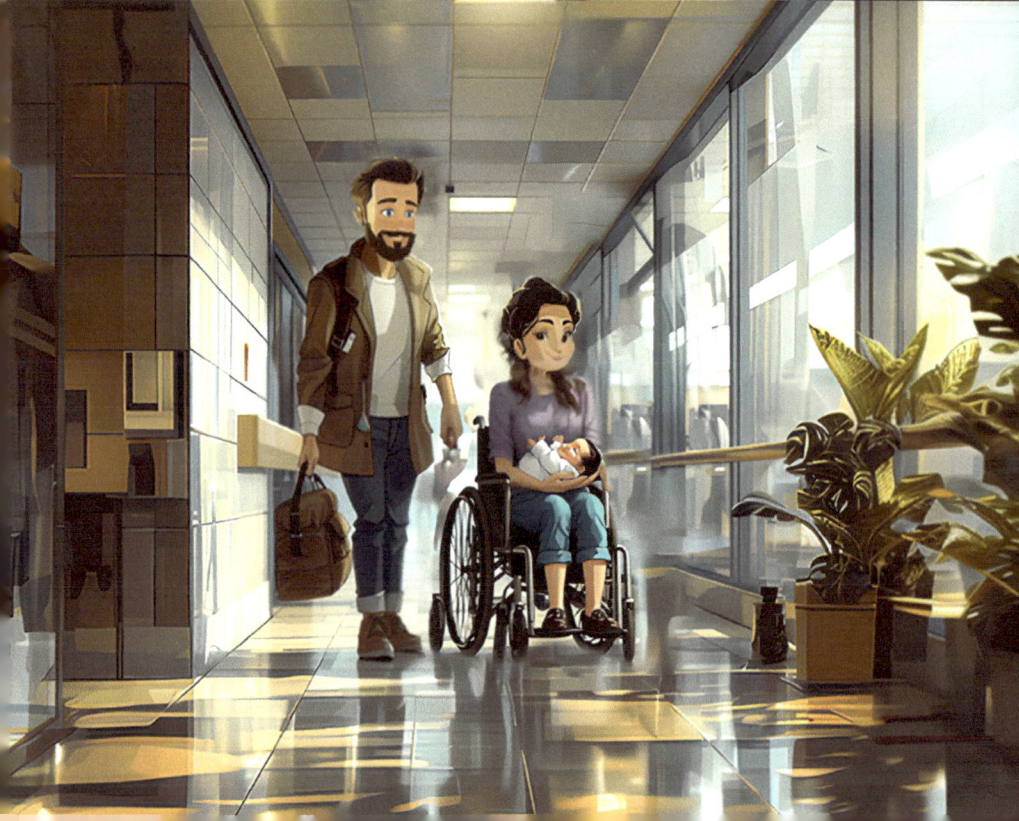
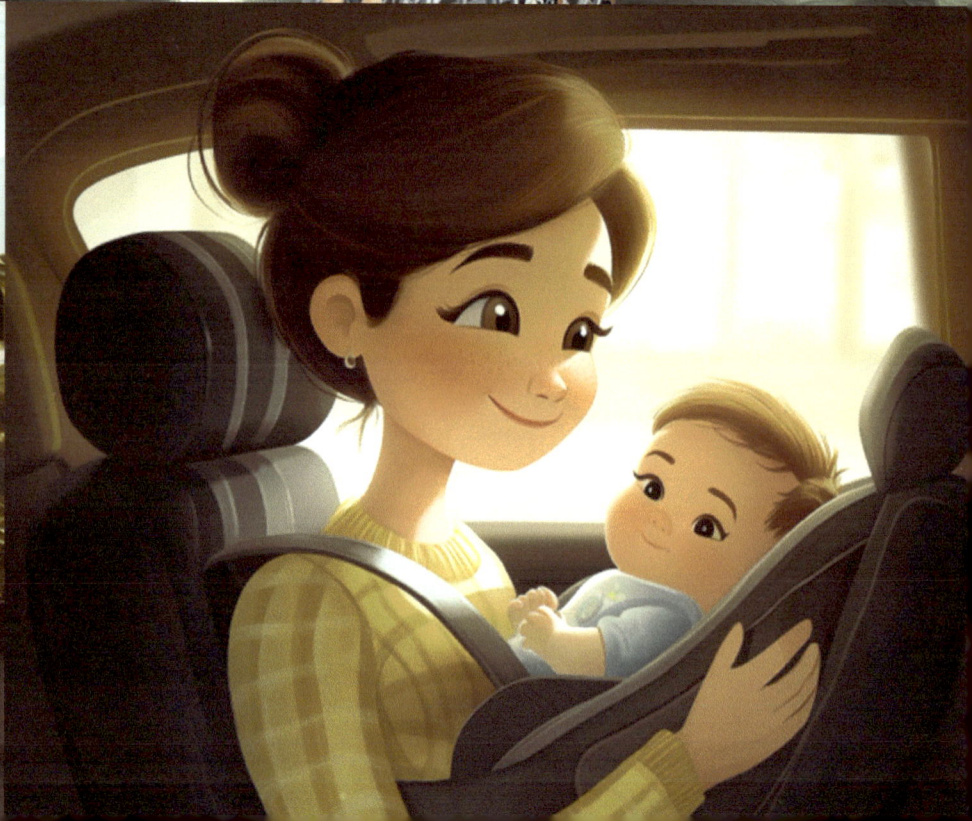

As the families left the hospital with their new babies in tow, the parents were excited about having a new little one to care for. Their thoughts included how they would provide for and protect their baby, manage their relationships, and how they might communicate with them as they grow.

The parents knew they would have many new experiences to prepare for along the way. For some situations, they felt prepared, and for others, not so much. But like all parents, they must consider ways to be flexible, supportive, and nurturing so their children will grow up with a healthy mind, body, and spirit. It may not always seem easy, but parents – like youth, have exactly what they need inside to make loving and supportive decisions as they move through life together.

Here are
some Nick Names
that people answer to

Pookie, Pumpkin, Sal,
Nikki, Ronnie,
Ro-Ro

YOUTH

Do you have a Nick Name or
Preferred Name?
What is it and Why?

ADULT

Do you have a Nick Name or
Preferred Name?
What is it and Why?

John, Mary, Donna and Daniel all had a nickname or a preferred name that made them feel confident about who they are as individuals. Nicknames, whether preferred or chosen, are abbreviated or alternate names that convey uniqueness.

Nicknames are used for various reasons. Sometimes they are self-elected, like Don, from the original name of Donna. Sometimes, nicknames are used because someone struggles (currently or in the past) with saying an assigned name or title correctly. For example, a grandmother may be called Gammy by family and friends because a grandchild couldn't say, "Granny."

Sometimes, nicknames are assigned by family or friends because of a specific life experience. For instance, let's say a child falls into a sandbox and gets sand in their mouth, the family may then adopt the nickname "Sandy" for that child, or a baby that scoots before they crawl or walk might be called "Scoots" even before they can self-select an alternate name.

A preferred name is self-elected, conveying personality or identity. When a person does not identify or relate to a name assigned to them at birth, they may formally or informally use a name that best reflects how they see themselves. Preferred names are just as meaningful as nicknames – because they reflect how someone sees themselves.

Identifying
pronouns include

She, Her, Hers.
He, Him, His.
They, Their, Theirs.
Zie, Zim, Zir.

ADULT

What are your identifying
pronouns?
What is it and Why?

YOUTH

What are your identifying
pronouns?
What is it and Why?

Johnnie, Mare, Don, and Ella, like other people, use pronouns to communicate gender identity. Gender identity is how we organically feel on the inside despite our external body parts. Traditionally, gender identities have been defined as, male with masculine expression if you were born with a penis, and it was assumed you'd have a tough demeanor and be physically strong; or female with feminine expression because you were born with a vagina and it was expected that you would be gentle and fragile–and, there was no other option. But today, we know that there are variations in gender identity. For this reason, we talk more about communicating identity than ever before.

If we think about what the words masculine and feminine mean, it becomes clear that we can't clearly define them by the assignment of body parts alone. This is because some people born with a penis organically have a soft and gentle persona with compassionate beliefs and expressions. Some people born with a vagina are by nature physically strong and have an affinity toward independence and a "take charge" way of thinking, feeling, and behaving. In some instances, some people don't connect with masculine or feminine traits at all. And, even still, some innately connect deeply with a sense of both femininity and masculinity, in every sense of being. This is why it's important to make room for each individual's experience, and pronouns help us to do that.

For those who don't relate to or identify with traditional gender expectations because of their DNA, hormonal structure, or personality, gender identity and expression may be non-traditional. The use of non-traditional pronouns helps to more accurately identify, and express identity to others. You may hear someone refer to themselves as "they," "them," "theirs" or "zie," "zim," "zirs." These are called, "Gender-Neutral Pronouns." Gender-neutral pronouns more accurately reflect an individual's identity without consideration of physical, social, or cultural-gender roles and expectations.

There is no right or wrong here. What matters most is listening, learning, and making space for everyone to be who they are and not who we want them to be.

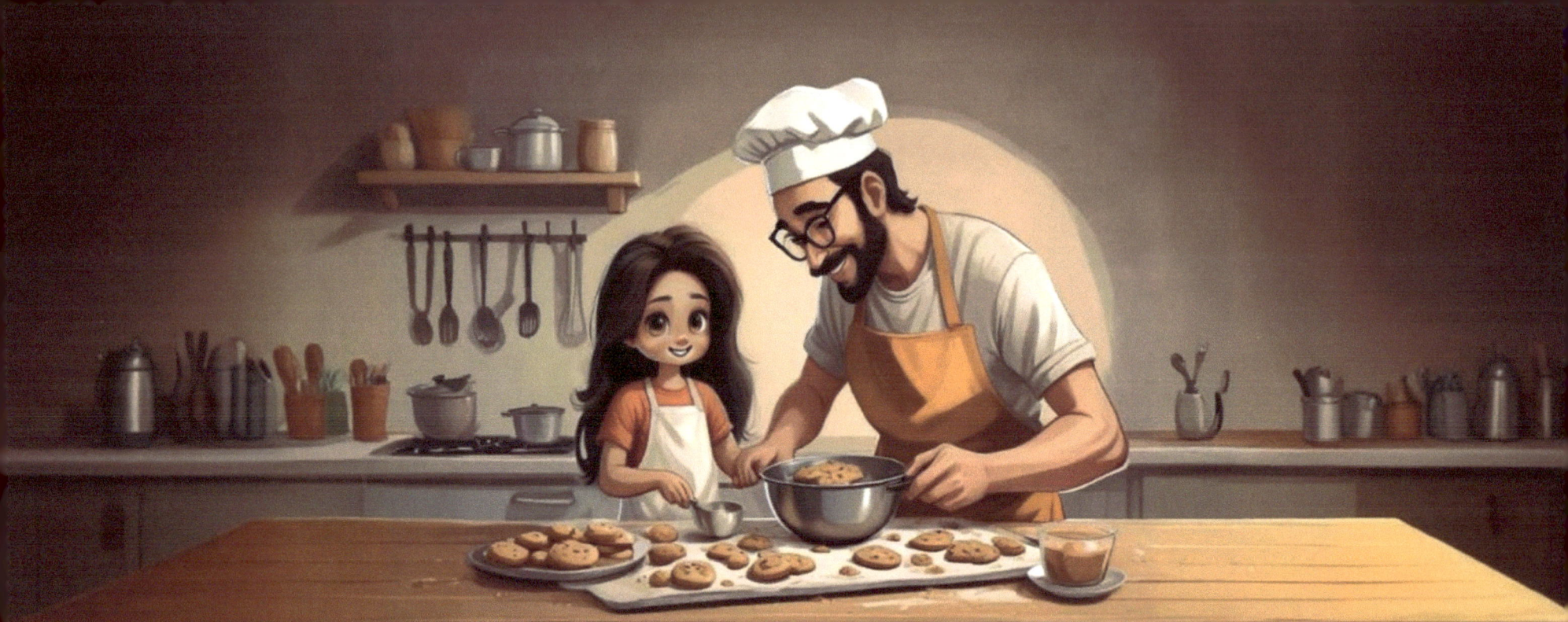

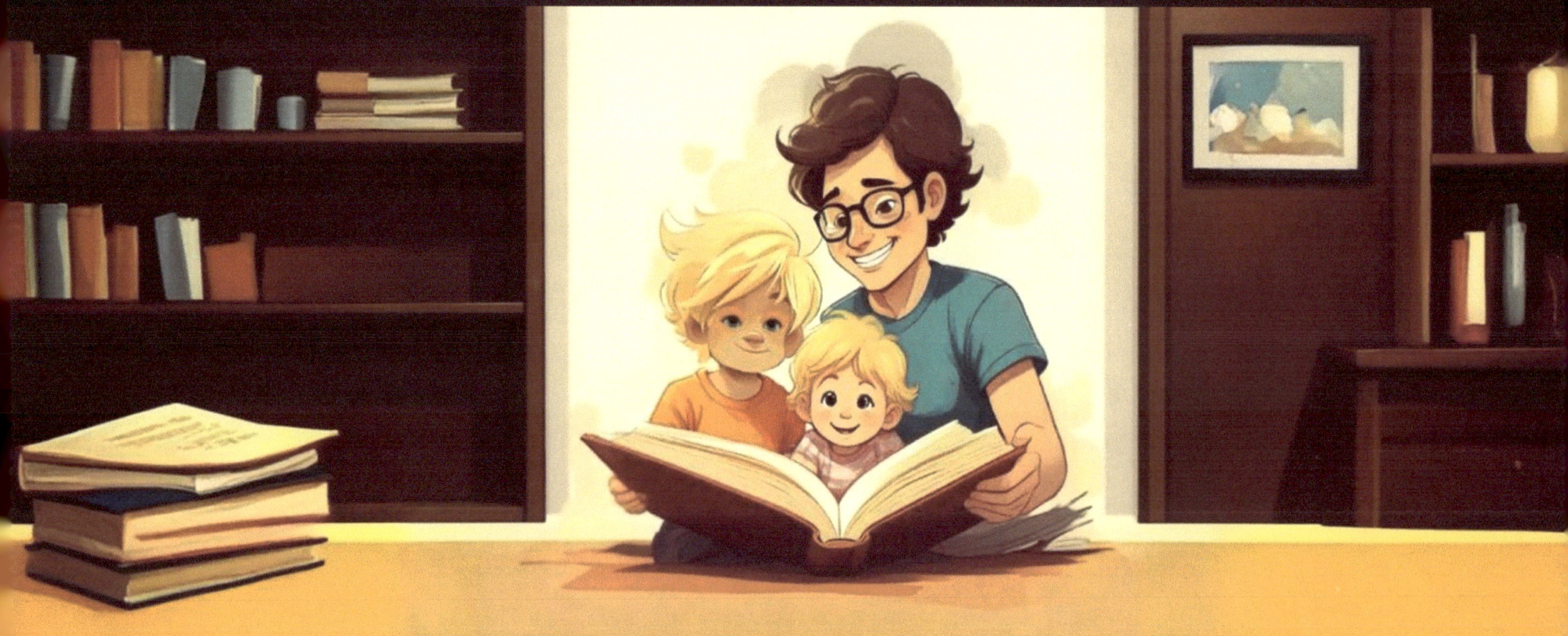

Talking about gender identity and expression can be emotional and sometimes difficult for both a child and their parent(s). Like the youth in this story, and children all around the world, every child needs to feel loved and accepted by their parents and caretakers. And, just like adults, youth need an environment of safety and flexibility to explore feelings and perceptions of self.

Parents can provide children with an emotionally safe environment to consider and explore gender identity and expression. This can be done by spending time together and facilitating communication that is open and flexible, allowing everyone to have their own thoughts and feelings. This would mean no one person's thoughts or feelings outweigh or overpower the others.

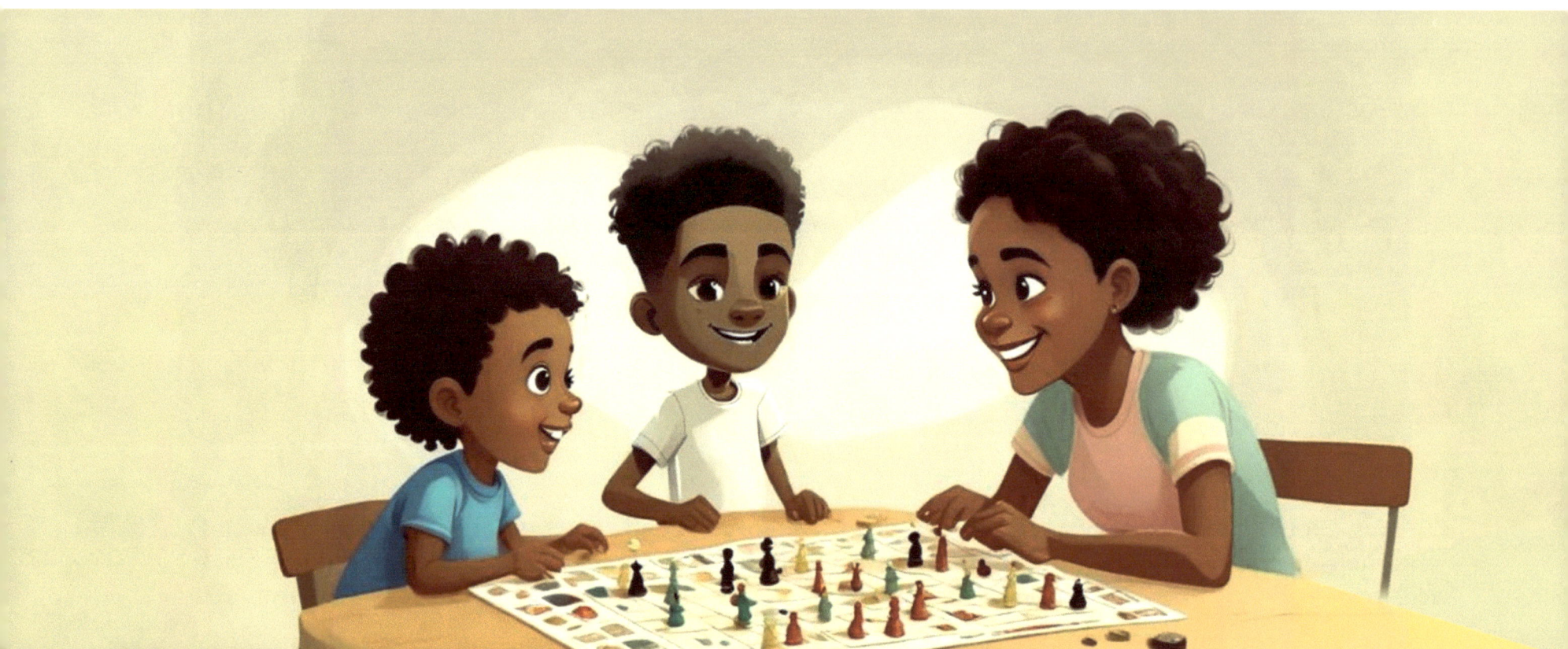

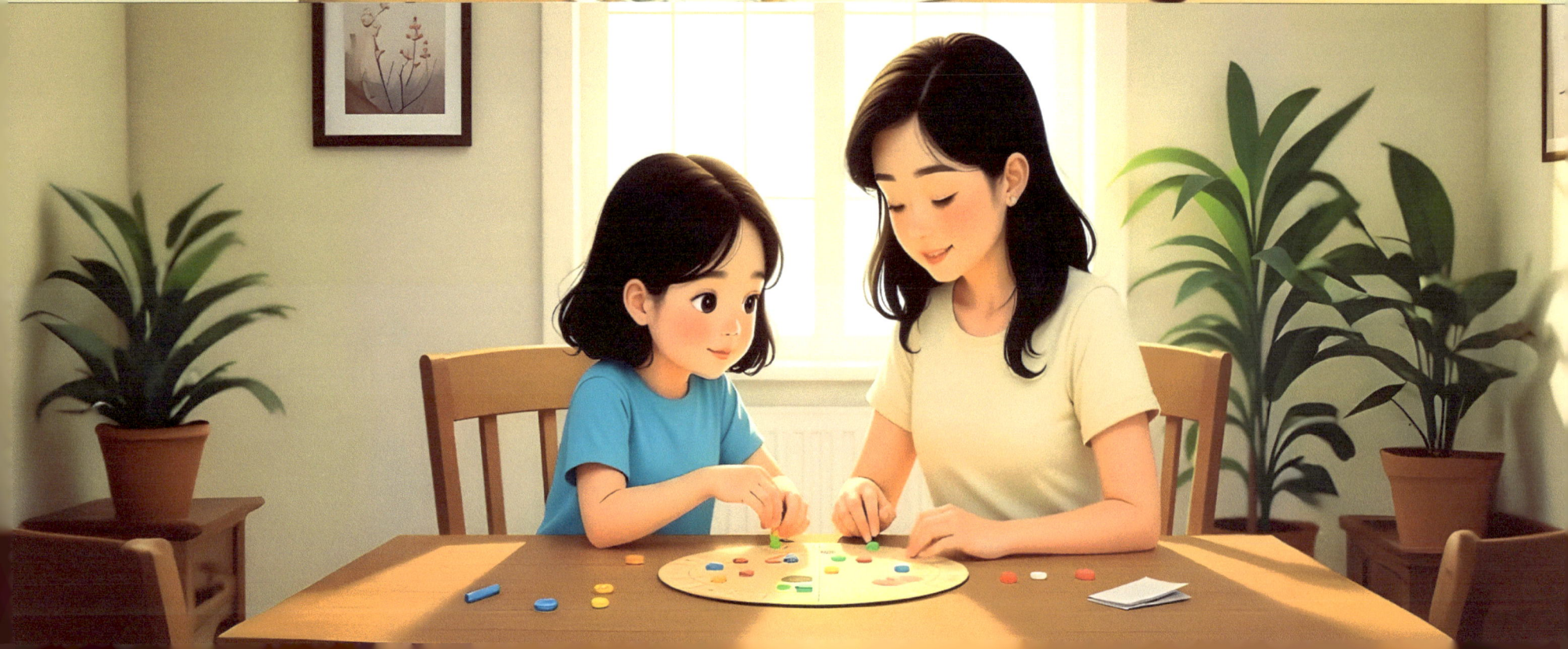

Conversations that happen with patience allow for the mental and emotional processing of benefits, potential consequences, or risks of one's thoughts, feelings, and actions. That's why emotional support from parents is so important. When parental support avoids the appearance of anger or shaming and does not promote guilt or harsh judgments, youth thrive. Emotionally safe communication between each parent and child regarding gender identity and expression enables both the parents and their children to develop and maintain a healthy awareness of self and relationship with each other.

So remember, in these conversations, connection matters more than perfection. And, what matters most is that you're staying engaged and present, even when things feel hard.

For All Readers of The Things Kids Learn Today: Gender Identity and Expression

Thank you so much for taking the time to participate in this learning opportunity about gender identity. With this book, I hope to make uncomfortable conversations easier.

While working in Social Services for more than 20 years, I've learned that sexual orientation and gender identity (SOGIE) is an evolving topic because people are talking more. For parents, caregivers, and teachers, if you don't shy away from the topic, you may find that the children in your life already know about SOGIE. SOGIE is not just about being Gay, Lesbian, or Transgender. It is about how we identify as individual human beings — each of us with our unique perceptions and life experiences. SOGIE-focused discussions take bias out of social and cultural expectations and allow us to be our unique selves as we identify with the world around us both spiritually and naturally.

I want to encourage adults and children to be open to respectful expressions of self, from yourselves to your children (if you're a parent or caretaker), fellow students and teachers (if you attend or work in a school setting), neighbors, and colleagues. Making room for self-expression is the same as making room for common courtesy. Respect, patience, kindness, and consideration are always appropriate in all relationships.

If you are not sure where to begin, there are lots of books, websites, television shows, movies, and support groups available to help you explore and have greater access to communication trends regarding gender identity and expression. If you are willing, you can begin to understand and observe the experience(s) of others, even if you are not comfortable with discussing your own SOGIE status. As you explore, you'll find the LGBTQ acronym has been expanded to reflect the wide diversity of identities and experiences, including those of allies. So, whether Lesbian, Gay, Bisexual, Transgender, Queer/Questioning, Intersex, or Ally (Straight), we are all in this together. We all have a right to Sexual Orientation, Gender Identity, and Expression because we are all uniquely made human beings.

For more information, see the Resources page of this book. And, wherever you are on your journey, you're not alone. Let this book and the resources included be the starting point toward greater understanding.

Resource Page:

LGBTQI+ RESOURCES

The following resources are available in the United States to support LGBTQI+ youth, families, and allies.

The Human Rights Campaign
https://www.hrc.org

PFLAG
https://pflag.org/about-us/

Strong Family Alliance
https://www.strongfamilyalliance.org/about/our-mission/

The Trevor Project
https://www.thetrevorproject.org/resources/article/friends-family-support-systems-for-lgbtq-youth/
and
https://pronouns.org

www.ingramcontent.com/pod-product-compliance
Lightning Source LLC
Chambersburg PA
CBHW041225020426

42333CB00004B/61